Hope after a Stroke? Yes!

Hope After a Stroke? *Yes!*

There Can Be Life after a Stroke, even a Good Life!

Wakie Trudeau McBride

TABLELAND PRESS

Copyright © 2025 Wakie Trudeau McBride

Hope after a Stroke? Yes!: There Can Be Life after a Stroke, even a Good Life! written and illustrated by Wakie Trudeau McBride

All rights reserved. No portion of this book may be reproduced, stored in a retrieval system, or transmitted in any form or by any means, mechanical, electronic, photocopying, recording, or otherwise, without written permission from the publisher.

Published in the USA by

TABLELAND PRESS, LLC
www.tablelandpress.com
info@tablelandpress.com

ISBN: 978-1-949323-16-0 (paperback)
ISBN: 978-1-949323-17-7 (ebook)

Scripture quotations are from the Authorized (King James) Version.

Book Cover Design by 100 Covers

Printed in the United States of America.

Dedication

I wish to dedicate this book to all of the people who were instrumental in my recovery in some large or small way.

To my family, for their love, patience, prayers, and the hundreds of ways they would drop everything to come to my aid. They supported me and encouraged me all along the way in every way they could and at any time of the day or night.

To the doctors and nurses, the many therapists (including physical, speech, occupational, massage, and lymphatic fluid drainage), and the doctors who recommended the different therapists. I can hardly leave out any one of the them. They all helped me so much.

To all my friends who were so faithful to pray for me and to cook and invite me to a meal with their families. They took me places I couldn't drive, especially to church. They wouldn't let me quit singing in the choir, even got me to start painting again when I couldn't even hold the brushes right or put them where I meant to put them on the canvas. They were such a dedicated bunch of friends and family.

Contents

Preface ix
Acknowledgments xi

1. Contributors to My Stroke 1
2. How My Day Went the Day of the Stroke 3
3. My Assessment 9
4. Depression 11
5. My Finances 13
6. The Turning Point 16
7. The Struggle 18
8. Painting Again 21
9. God Answers Prayers 24
10. The Courtship 26
11. I Was So Embarrassed 28
12. My Life with John 30

13. My Present Life	35
14. Twenty-Four Years after the Stroke	38
Appendix	45
About the Author	49

Preface

There really can be a happy and fulfilling life after a devastating stroke. I had been enjoying my life and the direction my life was going until my husband Jim's death in July 2000. I had spent a lot of time studying art and about thirty years giving art lessons. In fact, I still had been giving lessons in my art and gift gallery in Sallisaw, Oklahoma, when I had the stroke in August 2000.

One Friday after lunch, Jim had called me at my gallery to take him to the local hospital. They life flighted him to Tulsa from there. He was dead on Monday morning.

I thought my life was rough, going through all of that. We had been married almost thirty years. I was just putting my life back together when I had the stroke, one month and one day later.

There are some classic symptoms that are usually present and recognizable. Slurred speech is the most common one. One side of your mouth drooping is another. Of course, if you are not looking in the mirror, you won't notice this one.

You may not have had the same type of stroke that I had, and may not have reacted to it in the same way as I did. This is the way my stroke happened and the way I responded to it. There was one symptom I recognized: My speech was garbled. I was rushed to the hospital, and the medical staff that was on duty that day told me I had had a stroke.

Hopefully, there is someone with you because you will not remember much of anything that is said or done that day. You may not remember how you got there, or why you are there, or much of anything for a week or two or longer. Or you may show signs that you are getting better. I would take that as a good sign. Maybe it was just a TIA (transient ischemic attack) and would soon be alright.

I hope this book helps you or someone you love. May God add his blessing to your life as you read this.

Acknowledgments

I want to thank Dr. Chang for recommending massage therapy and lymphatic fluid drainage therapy. I am still in both of those.

I wish to thank a special therapist, Eli Mead, PT, DPT, who worked so gently on my ankle to get it more mobile. I feel that that round of therapy was the beginning of my getting the feeling back in my foot and leg.

I want to thank my church families for all the prayers and support, especially Ewell and Kathy Adams, Jim and Debbie Sparks, Deborah Brayboy, Georgia Heatherington, and Mary Beth Mattox. Some people just go above and beyond all we could ever hope for.

I thank my mom and dad for instilling in me such determination and grit, which makes you stay in there and just keep on fighting.

I hope I have not stepped on anyone's toes or left anyone out who has helped me.

Chapter 1

Contributors to My Stroke

At the time of my stroke, I was mourning the death of my husband, who had died with very little warning. I was also sleep deprived. Jim had had sleep apnea, but he couldn't use the CPAP machine. I had learned to sleep when he was snoring because I didn't worry about him as long as I could hear him. When he would stop snoring, I would awaken and shake him so he would breathe. I had this thing called "sleep habits" down to a fine art: Sleep when noisy, wake when quiet.

After Jim's death, I couldn't go to sleep in our bedroom because I would wake to every little sound. I would go back to the den and watch TV until I would fall asleep in the chair. Then I would go, half asleep, back to bed.

There were several other things that contributed to my stroke. I was not eating well and not taking good care of myself. Also, I was worried about my finances.

I was an artist, a businesswoman, a Sunday school teacher, a grandmother, a landlord, and the legal guardian for a disabled veteran. I was also holding drawing and painting classes at the art and gift gallery and frame shop that I owned and operated.

I had closed the gallery because of Jim's death and had just opened again for business. Then, just one month and one day after his death, I had a stroke. And everything stopped.

Chapter 2

How My Day Went the Day of the Stroke

The day leading up to the stroke started like any other day. Little did I know that my life was about to change for the rest of my life. This may be helpful to you to recognize the symptoms of a stroke. I didn't recognize them as quickly as I should have.

I had an appointment about thirty miles from my home in Sallisaw, Oklahoma. I drove to Poteau, Oklahoma, the closest Social Security Office. I got there on time. No problem. We finished on time. No problem.

Then I drove a few miles to my sister Vickie's home to have lunch with her. After lunch, I told her I was so sleepy I couldn't drive home without a nap (symptom #1). I didn't recognize it as a symptom. I took a nap, then got up, and drove home. I ran off the road three times (symptom #2). I still didn't get it.

When I got home, the first thing I wanted to do was (you guessed it) take a nap. I just thought I was that tired (symptom #3). Missed it again. I was awakened by the postman's ringing the doorbell. This is one of the things I like about living in a small town: Everyone takes care of each other, especially when there has been a death in the family. There was a life insurance check in the mail, but it was for several thousand dollars less than I had expected.

I called the insurance agent who had filed the claim on Jim's insurance. He said he would take care of it for me if I would bring the check to his office. On the way, my right foot began to go into a hard cramp, so much that my toes pulled down (symptom #4). Missed it again. I thought, *This shouldn't be possible. I'm wearing an orthotic in that shoe.*

When I got there, the agent found that Jim had been drawing a dividend check on that policy. I started to say thank you to the agent and realized my speech was garbled. Finally, I got the message! I suddenly thought, *I'm having a stroke.* Then I very slowly and carefully said, "I . . . think . . . I . . . am . . . having . . . a . . . stroke."

I started praying silently as the agent got me to the hospital quickly. Timing is so critical, and I had already wasted almost all day! The medical staff has just a short time to start treatment. If I had only recognized any one of the symptoms sooner.

On the way to the hospital, I remember thinking,

I've got to keep my mind busy. I've got to connect and think. I would repeat in my mind the names of my brothers and their wives, then my sisters and their husbands, then their children in birth order. You may not think this is important, but, believe me, if you have had a stroke, it is not only important, but very difficult.

At the hospital, I was given a quick examination and a CT scan to check for bleeding on the brain. Then, I was told I had had a stroke and was given an aspirin. My daughter, Sherry, was there before I was dismissed. I was sent home without a prognosis or any instructions, that I remembered. There are a lot of things that I do not remember during that day and for many days afterward.

In a matter of hours, I was almost helpless. I just wanted to sleep all the time. By the next day, I was much worse. My right foot and hand looked deformed, but try as hard as I could, I could not straighten them. They were in the hardest cramp I had ever had. Sherry took me back to the hospital, but they didn't do anything.

The following day, she called Dr. Rick Robbins. He examined me and confirmed the stroke. He prescribed a blood pressure pill and told me to take an aspirin a day. The doctor also said that I had a lesion in the back of the brain. He told me it may clear up in a few days. Well, it didn't.

The next day, on that doctor's orders, I was given an echocardiogram. Two days later, I had an MRI brain scan, a POB carotid Doppler ultrasound, and flu tests. I was given Clonidine (for what, I don't know), Zoloft for depression, and something for blood pressure. Sherry tells me that the doctor was very encouraging, but I do not consciously remember that.

In a few days, I was worse. I tried to keep my mind functioning. My brother Jack told me to dump the change out of my piggy bank, separate it by denominations, and count it. I was to put the money back, dump it out again, and start all over. I did that and everything else anyone suggested.

I was almost helpless. I couldn't sit up without falling to the right. I couldn't stand alone and couldn't walk without guidance. I dragged my right foot. Because my right toes were cramped under, I walked on the side of my right foot. I couldn't talk or even think of the words I wanted to say. Every time I got up, from sitting or lying down, I wet my pants. I couldn't feed myself either. It was evident I couldn't stay alone. At first Sherry stayed with me. Then my brother Jack and his wife, Jean, stayed two weeks to help me get around.

I fell a lot, maybe five or six times a day. The falling continued for about one-and-a-half years. I was very fortunate not to have broken any bones during that time. Or so I thought. I had to have my right foot and ankle x-rayed recently and was told that my foot and ankle had been broken many times. I guess, looking back, I just didn't have enough feeling in that foot, at the time, to realize that it was broken. My balance and coordination were still not very good.

At this point, the most important advice I can give you is to go as soon as possible to a neurologist, preferably one who specializes in stroke victims. Sherry tells me I saw one about four or five days after I had the stroke. That is part of the memory that was lost to me. What I do remember was sitting in a neurologist's office and wondering what I was doing there.

It is strange how the mind works sometimes, and other times it doesn't. You never know which it will be next. That's the reason you should get all the help you can as quickly as possible. A stroke is serious enough that you shouldn't waste time.

Medical professionals can examine and evaluate you. They can diagnose a stroke and can prescribe medication and therapy. However, they are not with a patient long enough at a time to fully evaluate the situation (in my opinion). This is not their fault.

They ask how we are, and we tell them we are fine. They want specifics; we can't give specifics. We can barely talk. Maybe we don't understand or can't think fast enough. Or maybe we are so thankful to be alive, we don't think to tell them how or what we are feeling.

Maybe they should push a little harder for more specifics. I don't know just how they could do this without offending. I'm not an expert on strokes and don't claim to be. The medical staff cannot understand how the patient feels because we don't tell them honestly how we feel. Also, they have not been able to walk through the progression of a stroke with the patient.

I'm going to give you exactly how I felt during the time that I was telling my doctor, "I'm feeling fine." This is my honest assessment, looking back on the situation as I see it now.

Chapter 3

My Assessment

I now began to assess the damage. Let's see. I can't walk. I can't talk or even think of the words I want to say. I can't even sign my name, and I have so many checks to write.

Sherry told me, "We will get through this together." She called the bank and told them what had happened to me in the last few weeks. They told her to write the checks and have me sign them the best I could. They would honor them.

I can't feed myself. I can't drive. I can't even use the phone because my mind won't work well enough to get the numbers right. In fact, the whole problem is my mind doesn't work right.

Also, the affected limbs (in my case, the right hand, the right foot, and the left side of my tongue) are in a hard cramp. So, nothing on the right side works right, if it works at all. I have even lost control of my bladder. I feel that I have lost my dignity and have lost my life as I knew it.

I lost my independence and ability to make

my own living. I had been an artist. When I lost the ability to draw, paint, and teach art, I lost my identity, what made me who I was.

I had my downtown art gallery to close. It was quite a blow to me. I could hire someone else to run it, but it wouldn't be the same. I was in no position to make the simplest decisions. Admitting I could no longer do what I was supposed to do, I decided to sell the gallery.

If you are lucky, you have lost the use of only one side. Hopefully, you will be able to use the other side more. I am right-handed and lost the use of my right side, but my tongue was paralyzed on the left side. If you can, use the hand that you don't normally use and really try to brush your teeth or your hair. Then, you can begin to understand a little.

Chapter 4

Depression

This is when the depression hits you. And it hits hard! You feel alone, lost, hopeless, depressed, and so utterly helpless. You cry and cry and cry. You want to give up. You want to crawl in a hole and stay there. But God isn't through with you yet. If He were, you wouldn't still be here.

For me, the depression was deep. It was the first time in my life I had ever been depressed. Now I could do nothing. I cried nonstop for weeks or even months. I do not remember how long this went on. It seemed like forever to me.

It is normal when you are depressed to think negative thoughts. However, there were many things to be thankful for. I could still breathe and didn't have to be put on oxygen. I still had my home. I still had my family, and they were very supportive of me.

I still had God's love, which I had through it all. Sometimes, His love was all that sustained me. I never prayed for healing because I had never known of anybody ever getting over a stroke. I did pray a lot for His help, and He helped me tremendously.

I do remember thinking I had imposed too much on my daughter, who had to work. I would go home with her in the evening and just sit and cry. This was not good.

For many nights after the depression began, I was not sleeping well. I called my granddaughter Christy and asked if she could come and get me. She and my daughter-in-law, Mary Jo, came by for me. They got something to help me sleep. After we ate the evening meal, I took the pill, and fifteen minutes later, I was asleep. I slept the whole night through.

After I saw the doctor again, he prescribed an anti-depressant, which helped a lot. At least I didn't cry all the time. I don't remember how many nights this went on.

Chapter 5

My Finances

After Jim's death, I needed to check on my finances to see where I stood. I knew I needed to know, but my mind was not working well enough. I had Sherry make a list of my assets and liabilities. I had her list all the credit cards, my balances, the amounts of the interest that each one charged, and all the other debts. I had Jack take a look at it, and he said, "It would take a miracle."

I made an appointment with a lawyer. I asked my son, Jim (I call him Doc), to take the lists to him and see if he could help me to decide what I could do. The lawyer wrote me a letter that basically said I would have to take bankruptcy. I had no other choice.

I asked Doc what effect it would have on the three houses that I owned jointly with my two sisters. He said they would have to go in the bankruptcy with the other property. I didn't have to think long about that. I couldn't do that to my sisters, or to the other creditors either, for that matter. I didn't file.

Instead, I asked God to help me out again. I went to my special chair I had been to so many times before to pray. I told God that I did not think it would be right for me to file for bankruptcy. Therefore, I would wait for Him to show me what to do or not to do. You may think I am crazy; you are not alone. While I was sitting in that chair, I fell asleep.

When I awoke, I had a clear plan that made sense to me. I got up and confidently began to set that plan in motion. First, I called the field representative for Kip, the veteran I was legal guardian for, and asked him if I could be Kip's principal caregiver instead of his guardian. He said no, he didn't think so. But he asked if he could come down that week for a personal interview with Kip and me.

During the interview, he said that after going over the records and having a discussion with his boss, they saw that in the twenty years that I had been Kip's guardian, they could find only about three dollars unaccounted for. The Veterans Administration not only made me the principal caregiver but also left me his guardian. That decision increased my income by nine hundred dollars per month. I planned his meals where I could handle them on time also. Part one of the plan had begun.

Jack had said it would take a miracle. It took

several, and my God, being the great God that He is, used several good and wise friends to guide me gently all the way. My best friend told me that her husband could help me with my finances. That's what he did before retirement. I asked him to help me, and he did. He took the list of my assets and how much income I could expect from them. If they were rental property, I could pay them off as we sold them.

Then, I could start with other bills and the credit cards. Another thing that I learned about the credit cards: Jim had one credit card in his name only, and it was maxed out. We called the company to tell them that Jim had died. They said they had to get his signature on the account first. We told them that they did not understand, that he had already died and been buried. They still argued, saying they would send their personal collection agent down and that he would have to produce that signature. Jack told them that after they had dug Jim up, if they could get him to sign their paper, good for them.

I went to my sister Pat's house for the weekend. She was an invalid, and I thought we could spend the weekend together, and at least, we could talk. On Monday morning I called my daughter to come get me. She came for me, and I got in the car, crying.

Chapter 6

The Turning Point

That was my turning point. I finally said, "I can't go on like this." Sherry took me back to the doctor, and he ordered some therapy.

When I went to the therapist, he asked, "Wakie, what did this do to your art?" I tearfully replied, "It completely destroyed it." He said they would put me in occupational therapy to get that restored.

I didn't believe the therapy would help. My dad had had a stroke and was completely paralyzed on one side until he died seven years later. He didn't really get therapy. A man came to Dad's house two or three times a week and massaged his hand, arm, and shoulder. Dad did not *do* his therapy. It was done to him. He did not put out any effort at all.

I did not just do the therapy when I was at the hospital rehab, but did it at home too. I was doing some kind of therapy throughout each day. Along with physical and speech therapy, I did all kinds of brain teasers, precision drawing, writing exercises, penmanship, sound and tongue exercises, and tongue twisters. I did stretching exercises too. I was doing some kind of therapy almost every hour I was awake.

From a stroke victim's viewpoint, I was retraining another part of my brain to do the things the now damaged part of the brain previously did. And it did work!

A few weeks later, I presented my therapists with pencil portraits of their respective families that I had done since I started the therapy. I wanted them to see the evidence that their therapy did what it was supposed to do.

Chapter 7

The Struggle

During the therapy, I began to make a little progress. After about six months, I was able to walk, with help, and talk (not plainly). My walking was still not very stable. My toes would still cramp under, so I was literally walking on the tops of my toes. I had walked on my toes so much that when they straightened enough, I had to have surgery on my toes.

Our living room was twenty-four feet wide. I would start walking across it with my toes cramped under. Then I would stop, stand still, and pray, "Lord, help me." I would then will my toes to straighten. With God's help, they would. Then I would take a few more steps. My toes would cramp again. I would stop and pray, "Lord, help me," and He would. And I would take a few more steps. Then I'd start all over again. This took much determination. But I aways was the stubborn one. I think that prayer, therapy, and determination are the keys to my recovery.

Another thing I did was to get tapes and CDs of old church hymns and try to sing along with them. The reason for using old hymns was that I knew the words from childhood. They were also an inspiration and encouragement to me. At first, I would be far behind because I couldn't form the words fast enough. Gradually, I got faster. Eventually, I was singing along with the hymns.

The stroke happened in August 2000. In 2002, just before Christmas, or two-and-a-half years after the initial stroke, I had an appointment with a neurologist after having a TIA. She ran many tests and put me on Plavix and Foltx, which is folic acid and B-complex. The doctor said it was good brain food, and I needed all of that I could get.

I have had several light strokes since that time and have had no lasting effects from them. The doctors assure me that there have been no more lesions in my brain. Every time I would have one of these mini strokes, I would get scared because they feel the same as a big one for a few hours. I would call my daughter, Sherry, when I had the first symptoms. If she could not get to me within minutes (she worked all over the state), she would call her brother, Jim (Doc), and he or some of his family would drop everything and be there in minutes.

Within three weeks of being put on the new medication, I laughed aloud for the first time in two-and-a-half years. Sherry and I were in the car together, and it made us so happy. That same week, my tongue was loosed from the grip of the stroke, so I could speak plainly enough to be understood. Also, I think my brain started functioning somewhat normally at that time. I continue to improve daily, and with God's help, I will continue to heal.

My recovery seemed to come in spurts after a round of physical therapy. The therapy would be for one thing, and that particular area would improve. But other areas would improve as well. My life would be easier after every session. No matter what the therapy was intended for, it always had results in more than one area.

Chapter 8

Painting Again

A friend then challenged me to do a painting for her. She said she wanted me to paint a portrait of her bird dogs. She didn't care if it wasn't perfect, but she wanted my first painting after the stroke. I just knew I couldn't do it. She said she knew I could. I still couldn't put my brush where I wanted it to go, and I did not want to do it. I didn't want to sign my name on a painting that I knew from the start would be sub-standard. I told her no and put her off as long as I could.

I finally set up a canvas and just stared at it. For about a month, I looked at that blank canvas. I was scared to death to get started. Her persistence finally won out. I got my paints out and got started, slowly at first. I started with the sky. That went pretty well. A lot better than I thought. So, I tried the distant trees. I was gaining courage. I finished the painting! I was ecstatic, and the client was thrilled too. There was no stopping me now.

My paintings took on a new dimension. The

floral paintings had a new brilliance. The animals had a new sparkle in their eyes. The landscapes were more realistic. One of my clients told me it was like I was seeing everything with a new insight and clarity. I sure do appreciate my friend's insistence. I was now painting again and loving it.

I even started teaching art lessons again and loved every minute of it. I loved seeing the excitement on the students' faces when they were learning something new.

I am including a print of the large painting, *Comin' at You*, thinking it may be an encouragement to you. The stroke happened in the year 2000, and I did the elephant painting, *Comin' at You* in 2003. I painted the elephants very large, 5 feet by 4 feet, in celebration of getting my faculties back. I have done more than forty paintings since the stroke. I sometimes feel like I should classify my art: BS (before the stroke) and AS (after the stroke). I owe that friend so much for jump-starting me.

[Note: Prints of *Comin' at You* are available on canvas or paper. Contact Wakie McBride at wakiemcbride@icloud.com.]

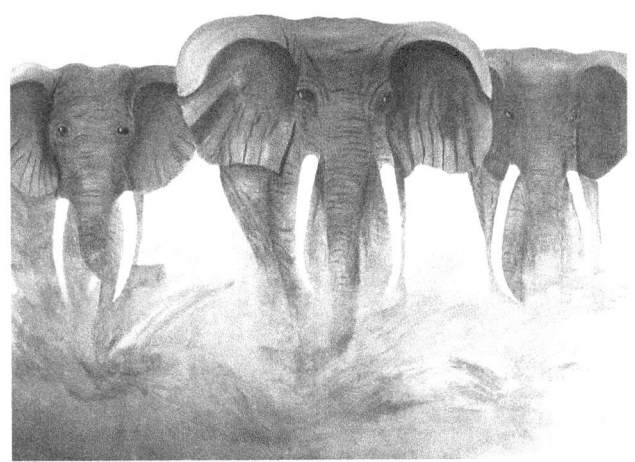

Comin' at You, oil

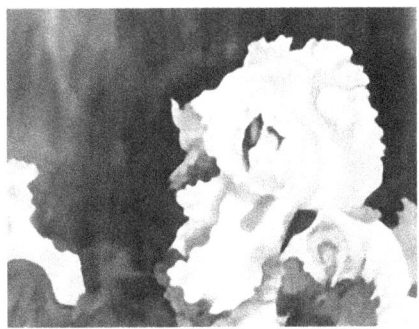

Before the stroke

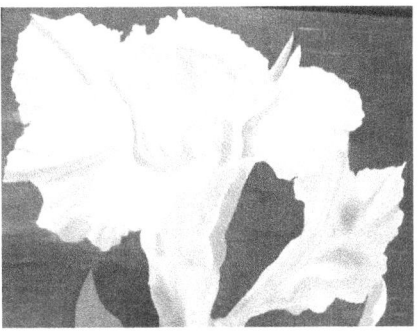

After the stroke

Chapter 9

God Answers Prayers

I was mentoring a young Christian lady, and I asked her if she would pray with me that if God had someone that He wanted me to spend the rest of my life with, would He show me and make it clear that He was leading. We had been praying for about six months, and this is what happened. God answered me again.

Sherry was living on the West Coast (California). And I had been visiting her and her family and had just come home. I was preparing to go to a Red Hat Society luncheon, when I got the feeling that I needed to go visit my brother Jack, who was living in Marietta, Oklahoma. But I argued with myself that I didn't have time. I had my classes to get ready for. They started Wednesday, and this was Saturday.

My brother Jack had not been in good health, and I thought, *He must need a visit*. So, I finally gave in. I started packing a few things. I usually took just casual clothes, but something or someone (now I know it was God) told me to take my best. I wondered why. *I must need to go to a funeral or something.* So, I took my best dress and shoes. I went to the luncheon, going east. Then I went west to visit Jack. You may have guessed: Jack and I were very close.

Jack and his good friend John McBride had both been in the Oklahoma Highway Patrol before they retired. They ended up living in the same town and going to the same church.

On Sunday morning Jack, his wife, Jean, and I went to church as usual. We sat down at the front as usual. When church was over, we got up to leave, and I looked up and saw John McBride coming down the aisle to meet us. Nothing unusual had happened yet. Since we are a hugging people, when we met, we hugged each other, exchanged a few words, turned, and walked to the back of the church as usual. Wait! There was something unusual about that walk. I realized that John and I still had our arms around each other's waist! This was unusual!

John told me later that he had been praying almost the same prayer for three weeks. His prayer was answered a lot sooner than mine, but what counts is that they were both answered! He also told me that he had heard a voice saying to him, "That's the one," when he first saw me coming up the aisle that Sunday morning.

Chapter 10

The Courtship

The next night, the pastor had a dinner at his home for all the seniors in the church. Of course, we were going. About thirty minutes before we left the house, John called to see if we were going. He asked if he could bring some ripe tomatoes before we left. We told him to bring them on. We all went to the dinner together, but in separate cars.

At dinner, my sister-in-law Jean and I sat at a table, while Jack and John sat at the counter. After we ate, as tables were being folded to be put away, John came up behind me and said something to me, but I could not hear him for all the noise going on around us. Besides that, he was standing at about six feet, and I was sitting at about five feet. So, I got up and asked him what he said. He asked if I had lunch plans for the next day, and I said, "No." He asked if I would have lunch with him. I told him, "I would be delighted." We went to lunch together the next two days.

He told me on the way to the restaurant that dating would be awkward for him because it had been over sixty years since he had dated. I replied, "It will be for me too." He said, "You should be aware, also, that a part of my heart will always belong to Ruby." (Ruby was his deceased wife.) I respected him for that. I replied that likewise part of mine would always belong to Jim.

That became evident later when one of us would call the other by our former mate's name. Neither of us was ever hurt by this. Instead, we rather felt honored, because we both knew that the other had never stopped loving their former mate. Their mate never stopped loving them—they died. There is a big difference between the two. The latter cannot be helped. It is not their desire to be absent from us.

I told him I had to go home the next day. We swapped phone numbers. He didn't call until Friday evening. I think we talked every night after that. He asked when I was coming to Marietta again. I told him I thought he should come to Sallisaw next. To that, his answer was, "When?" I said, "Anytime."

I went to my pastor and told him that I thought I had met my soulmate. I asked him to pray for us that God would lead us. He prayed and thanked God for John. John came the next weekend.

Chapter 11

I Was So Embarrassed

A few weeks later, John was coming again. I had invited my pastor and his family, and the music director and his family, and my best friend, Kathy, and her husband, Ewell, to meet John.

When the pastor came in, he asked if he could look at the studio. I didn't understand but said, "Sure." Introductions were made, and we sat down to dinner.

When the conversation started at the table, I didn't know what to think. First, the pastor asked Kathy if she thought the studio would make a good room for the boys. She said she thought it would. We didn't know what he was talking about. Then he asked me if I planned to take the furniture or leave it. I knew then he was talking about when John and I were married. Then he asked John when the wedding was taking place. John had picked up on it sooner than I had. He said, without hesitation, "In the spring."

Ewell saw my dilemma and came to the rescue.

He said, "You are getting the cart ahead of the horse. I don't think John has asked her yet." We all had a good laugh. They all loved John. And we changed the subject.

As soon as the rest of the guests were gone, John, laughing, said, "We had better make this legal. Will you marry me?" I said, "Of course."

The fact that we did not know was that missionaries from our church were coming home after five years on the mission field in Africa, and it was Kathy's job to find them a home. And the pastor thought they had found them one: mine.

Chapter 12

My Life with John

John and I were married the last Saturday before Thanksgiving; we didn't want to wait until spring. He was a very good man, and we were soulmates. We felt free to talk about anything. We prayed together and had our daily devotional time together.

He would come in the house from working in the garden or lawn. If I was taking the clothes out of the washer and putting them in the dryer, he would say, "Why didn't you call me to help you do that?" John was the kindest man I had ever known. When he had to go to Ardmore for something, we both went, holding hands all the way.

We were always together, unless John was working with his best friend, Joe. They worked together so well and were so close. Almost daily, they worked at the church. When they were not doing that, they were doing something for someone else in the community. It was their way to help the neighborhood. They loved their community and the people in it.

I had a TIA several years into the marriage, just before Christmas, and he was very supportive. He realized what was happening to me before I did and got me to the emergency room within minutes. I tried to talk on the way to the hospital, but I couldn't say what I wanted. I would start crying, and John would say, "You are going to be alright." Again, I kept my mind busy, but my speech would not come.

He took me to Mercy Memorial in Ardmore, Oklahoma. They went to work immediately with all kinds of help. Within minutes of our arrival, they had taken X-rays and a CT scan to check for bleeding on the brain and given me a shot to thin my blood and prevent clotting. They kept me there four days and kept me on a heart monitor and continued giving me shots in the stomach. I had no ill effects and was speaking within hours.

We were healthy and strong most of the time and were able to do a lot of things. Both of us enjoyed our life together. Our church meant so much to both of us. It was an extension of our family.

Our best friends had a motor home, and they went on a Volunteer Christian Builders trip each year. John had gone on one with them and had enjoyed it so much. We soon bought a motor home. That was about the first thing we bought together.

We went almost every year on the Christian Builders trip after that. We went on several other camping trips, either alone or with friends (sometimes as many as five motor homes together). There were about one hundred on the Builders trips, and they were considered our summer family, all one hundred of them.

John and I did a lot of volunteer work that John had already been doing. We were almost inseparable, and we were very happy together and enjoyed just being, no matter what we were doing. Our life was like we were young again and starting over.

We were happily married for almost twelve years before he departed this world. It was a very great loss for all of those who loved him, and that was all who knew him. John was sick most of his last two years, and we spent about as much time in the hospitals as we did at home.

I had a wonderful friend across the street, Marcie, and she told me early to not put John in the nursing home. She was a certified nurse's aide. She said that, together, we could take care of John at home. We did, with her doing most of the work, lifting him by herself most of the time. Joe, his best friend, helped a lot too. Many times, John would fall, and Joe would have to be called to help get him up.

John had always made a large garden, and he loved gardening. Joe parked John's riding lawn mower close to the door so he could get on it and ride around outside and keep his eye on the garden. We all worked together to help John enjoy his life as much as possible.

John flatlined several times in that last year. One of those times, he was hemorrhaging so badly it took a half day to get him stable enough to get him from the emergency room to intensive care. I was sitting beside his bed, holding his hand. He squeezed my hand and said, "Honey, if this is the end, and it seems it is, I don't want you to worry about me, because I will be in a better place. And I won't worry about you, because you are a wise woman, and you can take care of yourself. And you will be alright financially. You will have my full retirement and the home." Then he flatlined again.

Nurses and doctors came running from every direction. One tilted the head of the bed down, and one started squeezing the blood bag. I started to get out of the chair and out of their way. One of the nurses just lightly, but firmly, pushed me back down and said in a soft, kind voice, "You stay right where you are. You are right where you need to be." I sat down and went back to praying. John was able to go home in a few days. That was a very tough time for both of us.

We lost him in January, the worst loss of my life. He was such a sweet man and died so peacefully, leaning on Joe on his right and Marcie on his left. I was holding his walker. We were looking him right in the eye and knew the minute his spirit left him. But we knew he wasn't hurting anymore. I knew I had to go on without him. I didn't know if I could do that or not. I love him so much.

Chapter 13

My Present Life

But life does go on, somehow. I am ninety years old, and my health is pretty good for my age. I am over the stroke completely, except my right foot and leg, which are always swollen. I have not regained the feeling in them. I don't always know if I'm standing on my foot or if it is turned under. If it is turned under and I step on it, I fall.

Sometimes when I am brushing my teeth or hair, my right hand will go into a very hard cramp, just like it did when I had the stroke. Even when I'm drawing or painting, my hand still cramps.

I took some more physical therapy recently (2023). It straightened my right foot and ankle quite a bit. I am a big believer in physical therapy. May I say that it is important for you to work at it and keep working at it. It doesn't do you any good for someone to work your limbs for you. It is the putting out the effort that works.

Here are a couple of Bible verses that helped me a lot while I was recovering from my stroke.

"They that wait upon the LORD shall renew their strength; they shall mount up with wings as eagles; they shall run, and not be weary; they shall walk, and not faint." (Isaiah 40:31)

"Be still and know that I am God." (Psalm 46:10)

Since John's death, my daughter, Sherry, had been trying to get me to come to the West Coast so she could take care of me in my old age. She was very persistent, and she has a condition that keeps her from traveling. I felt it was the only unselfish thing for me to do. So, I gathered up everything I owned and sold it, said goodbye to friends, and called my friend Kathy and asked her if she was ready to go to California to help me drive. The next day we were on our way.

I have a good life now with Sherry, Doug, and Sarah, and enjoy being with them. They are such a sweet family and have gotten me some of the best medical help possible. I am very happy in my downstairs suite. We all get together downstairs for the evening meal and play some board games or Mexican Train, or just sit and talk. And we are together a lot of the time.

I have written and illustrated my first book,

Drawing for All Ages, under my pen name: Wakie Trudeau McBride. I completed it after John's death. It was released May 6, 2024, and is on sale at most online places that have books for sale. I enjoy the challenge of writing and am still drawing and painting. I haven't had the courage to teach. I don't think I have the stamina for it.

This is what I thought was the end of the story. But something else has happened that I must include. Here is the rest of the story.

Chapter 14

Twenty-Four Years after the Stroke

On August 13, 2024, almost exactly twenty-four years since I had the stroke, I awoke with feeling in my right foot. I could feel my big toe and the next one move. I not only felt them move, but I could move them for the first time in twenty-four years!

The next day I had an appointment with another doctor for an unrelated procedure. He told me the pros and cons of having it done. We both agreed to not have it done. Under my breath, I said, "Good, I didn't want to right now because I had feeling in my foot for the first time in twenty-four years." I didn't think he heard me. He came closer, squatted down right in front of me, and calmly asked, "What happened twenty-four years ago?" I repeated the story to him, and we talked about it for a few minutes.

And then he said, "I'll tell you what I want

you to do. I want you to get an appointment with a massage therapist, and I want you to keep me posted. I want you to tell me everything that happens to that foot." He said it as though he expected more to happen. He said, "I am a professor. And we are always learning and teaching, and teaching and learning. I want to know all about this." It was like he thought there's more to this story. I left his office so excited about maybe making a full recovery.

I was very fortunate. The therapist had a cancellation, and I got an appointment for the next day. Alicia gave me an hour massage. I told her that I had feeling in my big toe and the one next to it two days ago. She started there first. When she started, I felt something, but I couldn't identify it. I asked her what I was feeling. She said she was working on the first two toes, and the other three toes on that foot started twitching.

She started working her way up my leg, putting pressure on the outside of my leg. When she was about halfway up to my knee, I could feel up to the knee. Then, I could feel up to my thigh. Before the massage session was over, I had feeling all the way up to my hip.

The next morning I awoke to that foot feeling warm on the bottom. I quickly felt the bottom of my foot with my hand, and it felt warm to the touch also. The next time I felt anything was a feeling as if I had had a shot of novocaine that was wearing off and starting to come alive again. This happened once the first time. Then, it happened three times in one evening.

One morning soon after this, I awoke to my right heel itching. I started exercising more to assist in the healing process. I have had several sessions with the therapists and am having more feeling in that leg. It no longer feels like I am dragging someone else's leg around with me. It feels like it belongs to me now. It is a great feeling, after twenty-four years of feeling nothing, not even pain, within the foot or leg. I could feel it if you touched it on the outside but couldn't feel anything on the inside that I knew was from that leg. It just felt like I had this huge, heavy leg that was hard to maneuver, and it was not a part of me.

I realize now the real reason I did not know when I had broken my foot and ankle so many times before was that I didn't have enough feeling to recognize it being hurt that badly.

I am taking massage therapy about once or twice a week and lymphatic fluid drainage therapy, which is new to me. They massage the lymph nodes in a way that the lymphatic fluid drains from the extremities where it has accumulated over the years of being hurt over and over. Now it can flow more freely to other parts of the body, thus taking the swelling out of my right foot and ankle. This will make it feel more normal. I can hardly wait!

You may think that I am living in limbo, but

there is something new happening almost daily that gives me more hope that I will be normal again soon. I started recording my progress.

October 2024
Now we all have Covid. Will get back to you soon.

November 6, 2024
I had movement that lasted about one-and-a-half minutes in my right thigh.

January 2025
Christmas has come and gone, as well as New Years and Covid. I have gotten more feeling in my right leg, like it belongs to me. I can walk more normally than I have in a long time. I had to postpone my therapy because we all had Covid, and then for the holidays. I am anxious to get back to work on it and see what else we can expect. I have another appointment with the therapist in two days.

February 2, 2025
I started to get up out of my chair. I led off with my left foot, then I felt my right foot was turned under. I quickly corrected it and stepped on the right foot with my full weight. It was the first time in twenty-four years that I had enough feeling in it to know that it was in the wrong position and could act fast enough to keep from falling! Praise God!

I am feeling great! The right foot and ankle feel as good as the left almost all the time! I praise my God for that.

June 8, 2025
As I got ready for bed, I felt a burning sensation in my big toe and the one next to it. I took my socks off and discovered that I still had my support hose on (I wasn't supposed to wear them to bed). They were too tight around the toes. When I took them off, the burning stopped.

It is my prayer that this writing has been an encouragement to you. If you know anyone that has had a stroke, please put a copy of this book in their hands. It would have been so much help to have had something like this to hold onto, in those dark days, to help me to understand what was happening to me. If I can encourage one stroke victim to try as hard as he or she can for as long as it takes, then my struggle will not have been in vain.

We sometimes wonder why these bad things happen to us. I think, sometimes we are too busy, too selfish, too conceited, and too independent for God to have His rightful place in our lives. I know I was all of the above. But I would go through it again, if necessary, for the spiritual growth, the insights, and the humility that I have learned. It taught me to slow down and to take each day as a gift from God, which it is, and to be so thankful for it. It taught me not to take anything or anybody for granted. It taught me just how fragile I am and how precious life is. It taught me that I cannot do everything, and that is alright. Everything is not about me, my wants and schedule, and that is alright too. We were meant to serve and to help others along the way.

Don't be afraid to lean heavily on God. He knows what you are going through. And He can handle it for you or through you or even in spite of you. Ask Him, and wait and see how He works. You will be so surprised.

Appendix

Disclaimer

I am not a medical doctor nor a member of the medical profession, nor do I claim to be. I am only a victim of a stroke, trying to give hope to other stroke victims by telling them about the stroke that I had and my response to it. I have almost completely recovered from the stroke. It has not been easy and has taken lots of prayer, stubbornness, and pure old-fashioned grit. But I was successful because I was determined to follow all of the instructions the therapists taught me to do. I had the stroke twenty-five years ago and am still recovering. I am thankful for everyone who has helped me along the way. Most of my doctors have been very kind, encouraging and very professional.

Symptoms that I remember (not meant to be a comprehensive list):

- Drooping on one side of the mouth
- Garbled speech (This may be the only symptom or the first symptom that you recognize.)
- Sleepiness

- Irrational driving
- Paralyzed hands, feet, or one side of your tongue
- Physically unbalanced (unable to stand up, stand alone, or walk)
- Unable to think of the words to finish a sentence

There are other symptoms that I have forgotten. I hope this helps you or someone you know.

Thank you for reading *Hope after a Stroke? Yes!* I pray that it was a blessing to you.

If you enjoyed it, please consider leaving a review on Amazon, Goodreads, or any other online retailer. Your feedback helps other readers discover new books.

About the Author

Wakie Trudeau McBride believes that part of the "art spirit" is to give back to the community and nurture emerging artists. For thirty years, she has taught art to all age groups in private classes and by special invitation in the public education system. She operated her own art and gift gallery for several years.

An accomplished artist and painter, Wakie has studied with Jim Fallier, AWS; Milford Zornes, Sheila Parsons, Larry Weston, Tony Couch, Lola Doom, and others. Having produced and sold over 250 paintings, she has had many one-woman shows and won numerous awards. She and her artwork were featured in *Oklahoma Artists of Distinction*. Galleries across the United States have embraced and sold her art. She has also exhibited at the Arkansas Wildlife Federation show.

She has been a member of several art associations, including the Sequoyah County Arts and Humanities Council (serving four different terms as its president), the Crawford County Art Association, the Goddard Art Center, and the Ardmore Art Guild. She also helped organize the Arts and Humanities Council in Sallisaw,

Oklahoma. Speaking on television or in person to numerous civic organizations, Wakie is an advocate for art as a way to create a balanced life.

In 2000, Wakie experienced a debilitating stroke one month after the loss of her husband. Finding herself unable to draw or paint, she did not give up. With prayer, occupational therapy, physical therapy, speech therapy, and a lot of determination, she began painting again. She started in oils because she had more time to think with oil than with watercolor, and the medium is more forgiving. Two and a half years later, she emerged more proficient than before the stroke.

Wakie wrote and illustrated *Drawing for All Ages* to continue sharing her love for art with more people. Her clear illustrations, beautiful paintings, and helpful instructions make drawing fun and easy for anyone wanting to learn to draw.

Also by Wakie Trudeau McBride

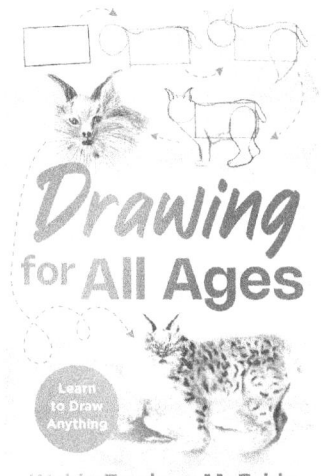

Wish you could draw? Explore eye-opening tricks to get started and simplify the process for a lifetime of enjoyment. If you or your child like knowing why as well as how, telling stories through pictures, and capturing your imagination on the page, you'll love Wakie Trudeau McBride's delightful doorway to developing your artistic eye.

Available on Amazon at
https://www.amazon.com/Drawing-All-Ages-Learn-Anything-ebook/dp/B0CZ7JYRY8

Sign up for the TABLELAND PRESS newsletter

and receive this FREE ebook!

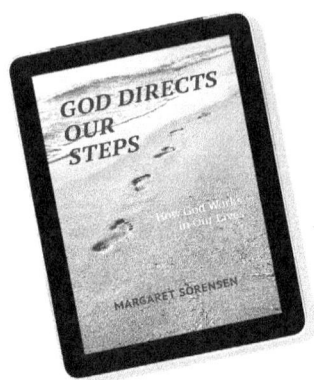

God Directs Our Steps – Discover how God works in your life by exploring how He directed the paths of eight biblical people.

Each month you will receive the latest news on upcoming books, plus devotionals, Christian book reviews and Bible quizzes.

Download your free PDF
of *God Directs Our Steps*
at www.tablelandpress.com

You Might Also Like

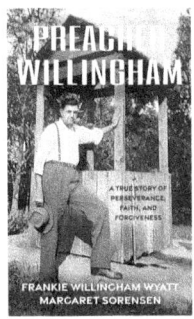

Preacher Willingham – Kidnapped as a baby and beaten as a child. Discover how Wesley Frank Willingham turned a childhood filled with hardships into a life of victory that glorified God.

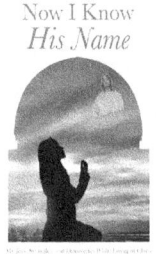

Now I Know His Name – Follow the adventures of Frankie Wyatt, a sixty-two-year-old widow, who answered God's call to share the gospel in China.

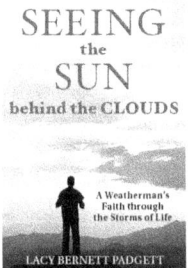

Seeing the Sun behind the Clouds – Learn how one man's faith sustained him, even when a medical crisis resulted in two below-the-knee amputations.

Learn more at www.tablelandpress.com.

www.ingramcontent.com/pod-product-compliance
Lightning Source LLC
Chambersburg PA
CBHW050045080526
44586CB00014B/1459